The Candida Remedy:
Cure Your Candida Yeast Infection And Lose Weight The Natural Way With This Easy To Use Guide

by Linda Shaw

Disclaimer / Limitations of Liability

Also by Linda Shaw:

Diary Of A Candida Sufferer: A Personal Journey Back To Health

To my husband Jeff, my rock during my years of suffering from candida overgrowth syndrome, then cheering me on and encouraging me during my healing. You have more than lived out your vow to be with me "through sickness and in health".

I love you.

Contents

Introduction

If you bought this book you have probably done enough research to conclude that you are suffering from symptoms of candida overgrowth, and you need help but are too overwhelmed with all the information out there to even know where to start. I know how you feel! I've been there too. Now my health is back and I feel great, but only after years of research and experimenting to develop the treatment plan I successfully used for myself, that I am now sharing with you. I have structured this book to be an easy to follow, step-by-step guide for you, with helpful tips and checklists to help you get started right away. This book is about using all-natural ways of healing with diet, supplements, self-care and lifestyle recommendations. I am not a doctor nor do I have any kind of medical degree, but the information in this book is what I learned from my own personal experience. Even so, I *urge you to discuss this plan with your doctor* before you start, especially if you are currently taking any medications and/or have any dietary concerns or limitations. Every body is unique, and though this plan worked perfectly for me, you may need to adjust it to fit your own unique needs or as recommended by your doctor.

I know you are eager to get down to the business of getting your health back, so I'll briefly touch on just what candida is and some of the symptoms of candida overgrowth. This information is easily found on the internet and I assume you have already done some research, which is why I won't spend a lot of time on it.

Candida is a yeast that we all have in our bodies, and it does serve a purpose. However, certain things will cause this yeast to grow out of control, like stress, poor diet, antibiotics, etc. Sometimes your symptoms will be only in a certain area, like vaginal yeast infection. Or, you may have system-wide issues like sinus infections, dandruff, digestive issues, hormonal imbalance, and even depression to mention a few. There are so many issues caused by candida overgrowth that are also caused by other disorders that it can be difficult to know if candida is truly the cause. A good rule of thumb is that if you have any of these symptoms and you have ever taken antibiotics, odds are you have candida overgrowth. Even more so if your diet consists mostly of fast foods, processed foods, refined carbs (white breads, rice and potatoes) and sugar.

Personally, I suffered from over 20 symptoms of candida overgrowth throughout my body, caused by stress, too many rounds of antibiotics and poor diet choices. Ironically, the antibiotics I took for my sinus infections were helping to cause the candida, which caused my sinus infections! And my sugar addiction was only made worse by the candida which, because its main food source is sugar, only made me crave sugar more. Today ALL my symptoms are gone, and I have had a passion for spreading awareness about candida overgrowth ever since. With this book, I am hoping to help others who are suffering with an easy to follow, all-natural plan that works.

10

Chapter 1 – Diet

I would have to say that the most important thing you can do to treat your candida overgrowth is to change your diet. See the handy Candida Diet guide starting on page 15 for the full plan. Basically what you want to do:

- Adopt a low-carb, no yeast, no sugar, whole organic foods diet.
- Eliminate sugar or get it down to no more than 5 grams per day.
- Become a label reader, make sure there are no preservatives and chemicals in the ingredients.
- Eliminate anything with yeast or made with yeast, like breads and anything with vinegar in it.
- Avoid fermented foods, like pickles and sauerkraut, as they are fermented with yeast.
- Avoid eating all fungi (mushrooms).
- Even fruit should be avoided during the healing phase, as it contains sugar.
- Also avoid alcohol, especially beer and wine.
- Stick with organic veggies and high-quality organic meat and eggs and you can't go wrong.

Stay on this diet for at least 3 months or up to 6 months, depending on how strictly you follow it, to completely cleanse your system of the excess candida.

The diet is by no means easy, and is probably the most difficult part of treatment. But it is the *most effective* part. All of the other things help, and are important parts of your healing, but if you do not start eating the right foods and stop eating the wrong foods, you will not heal completely. I know this from experience. When I finally added the diet plan to my healing regimen, my health improved much more quickly and in a few short months most of my symptoms were gone. The bonus was that I also lost 20 lbs! Not a pound came off until I changed my diet.

Refined carbs and sugar *feed* the yeast you are trying to kill, as yeast loves sugar. It makes no sense to try to kill the yeast while feeding it at the same time. If you are used to processed, convenient foods that are full of sugar and refined carbs (which convert to sugar in your system), a candida diet will be a difficult transition at first.

After a couple of weeks, however, when the major part of your detox has passed and you are feeling much better, you will find your sugar cravings have ceased and you are starting to enjoy your new, healthy way of eating. You may even be losing weight, which really helps to reinforce your will power! Just be sure to find some recipes that you love and that are of course "legal". Organization and preparation are key, especially if you lead a busy life.

Some tips: Pick a start date, typically the next Monday. Put together a meal plan for the week. From that, make a shopping list and get all that you need, and then prepare all of your meals ahead of time for the week. If you have your special foods available for you all week, you will not be as tempted to eat junk. Portion out your meals and snacks in baggies and plasticware so you can quickly grab what you need for the day. Keep a written meal plan handy to stay on track.

On the proceeding pages is a handy diet guide for you to use to help you stay on track. This guide was my Bible when I was in my healing phase! I admit I was not 100% strict, so that is why it took me five months to get through my healing phase. It's up to you how quickly you arrive at the other end of your healing, with weight lost, a clear mind and a healthy body. Just stick with it, take it one day at a time, get back on the program if you slip, and you won't regret it! It is worth it. *You* are worth it!

CANDIDA DIET - Healing/Weight-loss Phase
(3 months if followed strictly, 5-6 months if not followed as strictly)
This diet eliminates sugar and any foods that contain sugar, yeast and anything made with yeast (such as many fermented foods) and foods that may contain mold (such as cheeses).

Each meal should contain about 2/3 protein and 1/3 complex carb.

PROTEINS
All red meats (grass fed organic) - 6 to 8 oz/day max.
All poultry (free range organic) - 6 to 8 oz/day max.
All fish and shellfish - wild caught only
Eggs (from organic free-range vegetarian-fed hens) –
4 eggs per day max.
Avoid:
Processed meats (like lunch meat and bacon)
Cheese of any kind (contains milk and maybe mold)

FATS
Extra Virgin Coconut Oil
Macadamia nut oil
Extra Virgin Olive Oil
Butter (organic)

VEGETABLES
All vegetables *except*:
Avoid:
White potatoes
Beets
Peas
Carrots
Tomatoes
Corn

GRAINS - 1/2 Cup cooked 1x/week as a group

Pastas
Brown rice pasta only

Whole Grains
  Brown rice
  Millet
  Oats
  Buckwheat
  Quinoa
  Amaranth
  Spelt

Breads - 1 slice/week
Yeast-free and whole-grain:
  Sourdough
  Rye
  Spelt
  Ezekiel

Cereals - whole grain & 0-2 grams sugar max.
  Oatmeal (not instant)
  Brown rice
  Mixed whole grain
  Puffed millet
  Rice
  Wheat
  Quinoa
  Kashi

LEGUMES - 1/2 Cup cooked 1x/week
  Lentils
  Kidney beans
  Black beans
  Navy beans
  Peanuts

NUTS & SEEDS - 2 oz./day
  Pecans
  Walnuts
  Almonds
  Cashews
  Pumpkin seeds

Sunflower seeds

Macadamia nuts
Pistachios

Nut Butters (except peanut butter) - 3 Tbsp/day

EXTRAS
Olives (4/day)
Avocados (1/day)

PROTEIN BARS/SHAKES
Protein bars (as a meal replacement only) - 1/day max
OR
Protein Shakes (as meal replacement only) - 1/day max

CONDIMENTS/BUTTER/OILS
All spices
Butter - 3 Tbsp/day max
Macadamia nut oil
Mayonnaise/Mustard - 3 Tbsp/day max
Lemon juice - 4 tsp./day

BEVERAGES
Water (at least 2 bottles or 64 oz./day)
Soda - Diet only, 1x per week max
Coffee/Tea - 2 Cups/day max (or none at all)

DAIRY
Heavy cream - 2 Tbsp./day
Avoid:
Milk of any kind (due to sugar)
Half n half (has milk in it)

ALCOHOL
No wine or beer of any kind (due to yeasts)
If you must, vodka and club soda with lemon or lime wedge

FRUIT

No fruits of any kind (due to sugars)

DESSERTS

Desserts made with stevia
See Thin For Good cookbook or many "low carb" recipes

Diet Tips

> Choose organic veggies, grass fed beef, free range chicken and organic eggs from free range chickens as the main staples of your diet. Add a small amount of low-glycemic (slow digesting) carbs such as brown rice and sweet potatoes.

> If you have a sweet tooth, as a lot of candida sufferers do, try taming your sugar cravings with stevia, a natural sweet herb that you can find in both liquid extract or powder form at your local health food store or online (I use NOW brand stevia extract). Add it to your tea or other food or beverage in your diet that would benefit from a little sweetening. Do avoid artificial sweeteners, as they are not natural and are toxic.

> Use sea salt, spices and herbs in your cooking to add flavor, especially garlic which is a powerful natural antifungal.

> Cook with coconut oil, another powerful natural antifungal.

> If you love soft drinks and find they are very difficult to quit (like I did), you can make your own cold, fizzy beverage that is sugar-free and has zero calories! Simply add liquid stevia extract (to taste) and liquid caffeine (which you purchase

online) to flavored sparkling water. For an even healthier option, brew some flavored green tea, add the stevia, then pour over ice. For maximum effectiveness, try to eliminate caffeine altogether, as it can contribute to making you more hungry.

➤ If you must, you can enjoy an alcoholic drink *once in a while* (just make it a very rare occasion during the healing phase). You make it as minimally damaging as possible with careful choices. Vodka is lower in sugar than most alcohols, and club soda is low in sugar also. So, I recommend a vodka and club soda (or if you are at home, use sparkling water) with a lemon or lime twist, and a little stevia to sweeten if so desired. This drink will do the least harm to your healing. Just don't have more than a couple!

Diet To Do

____ Change your diet: think low/no sugar, low carb, no yeast, whole organic foods.

____ Use the candida diet guide and some recipes that you love.

____ Plan your daily meals and snacks every week.

____ Shop for your meal plans every week.

____ Read all labels.

____ Prepare/cook all your meals and snacks for the week. Portion out for maximum convenience.

Chapter 2 - Detox

The first thing you will start to notice when you change your diet is that the yeast will start to die off because you are starving it, and you will have detox symptoms. These symptoms will be the same ones you've been having, but at least this time it will be temporary, and not continual. You will have your good moments and then notice suddenly you have a headache, or your sinuses are acting up, or your digestive system is in an uproar.

Take heart my friend, this is actually a good thing. Your body is simply ridding itself of all the dead yeast and toxic build-up. Your body is designed to heal itself, and now that you are giving it what it needs to heal, that is what it is doing. Isn't that just amazing? Very soon you will be feeling better than you've felt in a long time!

If you work full time, see if you can take a week or even two weeks off work when you first start on this plan. You may not be feeling up to working while you are needing to visit the restroom or are having a detox headache or fatigue. If you are at home, you can care for yourself better during this part of the healing phase.

Here I will list the three major components of a good candida detox, as well as plug some products that I have used with good results:

Antifungal supplements. Some of the ingredients you would find in a quality antifungal supplement include garlic, olive leaf extract, oil of oregano and caprylic acid. I highly recommend the following brands:

- Garden Of Life Fungal Defense (includes beneficial probiotics)
- Zand Candida Quick Cleanse
- NOW Candida Clear

Very important *companion* supplements to the above are:

- Probiotics (a must for the gut!)
- Adrenal Support (with actual adrenal cortex – a must for fatigue!)
- Milk Thistle (helps the liver process the toxins)
- Fiber (helps move the toxins out)

For probiotics, I use Garden Of Life's Primal Defense. For adrenal support, I use Enzymatic Therapy's Fatigued To Fantastic Stress End. For my sensitive digestive system, I have found Enzymatic Therapy's Fiber Fusion to be the most effective. As for milk thistle, I have no preference. I usually get the least expensive brand I can find, as it works just as well. On the other hand, I would say "spare no expense" when it comes to the antifungal and probiotic supplements. There are many brands and blends of ingredients out there, so you will ultimately find what works best for you. These are just what I recommend in case you want to start quickly with some good, high quality supplements and go from there if needed. I particularly like

Garden Of Life products. They cost a little more than most, but the quality is excellent. If you have ever read GOL founder Jordan Rubin's story, you would appreciate why these supplements are of such high quality, and work especially well for those of us with digestive issues.

Sweating. Your skin is a major outlet for toxins. Help your body rid itself of toxins by working up a good sweat session at least 5 days per week. Three ways to do this (exercise sweat does not count):

1. Hot epsom salt bath (best done before bedtime)

   Make it hot enough so you start sweating after about 15 minutes, then stay in for at least 15 more minutes. Use a candy thermometer to get the water to the temperature you like. Use 2 cups epsom salts which help draw out the toxins. You may also use a few drops of essential oils like tea tree and lavender, which offer the bonus of aroma therapy and help your skin to stay soft.

2. Traditional Sauna

3. Infrared Sauna

Detox your life with natural cleaning and health & beauty products. What good would it do to be ridding your body of toxins, only to be slathering them back on in the form of commercial hair and beauty products, with all their chemicals? Not to mention commercial cleaning products! Here are ways to further your cleansing by extending it to your hair, skin and dental care, as well as cleaning:

- Swap out your shampoo and conditioner with organic shampoos and conditioners. I use Desert Essence hair products, especially the coconut shampoo and conditioner, which contain natural antifungal ingredients for your scalp.

- Use natural lotions, soaps and body wash products. I like Nature's Gate and Kiss My Face products.

- For your teeth, use a flouride-free toothpaste. I like Kiss My Face toothpastes.

- Ladies, use as much natural makeup as possible. I use Bare Minerals makeup.

- Also ladies, never use tampons or pads that have fragrance!

- When cleaning the bathroom, simply use water and a good microfiber cloth. You won't believe how easy it is to clean away scum with a microfiber cloth! Or you can make your own cleaning solutions using vinegar and baking soda. There are a few good all-natural cleaning products in stores also, even a natural disinfecting solution made by Seventh Generation that I use for cleaning the toilet.

- For laundry, use "free and clear" type detergents and dryer sheets. ECOS brand is a good brand. You could even make your own detergent!

Detox Tips

➢ Try rotating your antifungal supplements. For instance, take one brand for a week or two, then another brand for the next couple weeks, then another, then start over. Make a rotation schedule for yourself so you stay on track. Mixing it up helps to minimize the possibility of the yeast building up a resistance.

➢ Ladies, if you find that you still struggle with extra weight and fatigue a month or so into the diet and detox, you may want to have your doctor test your thyroid hormone levels, as hypo-thyroid (low) is not uncommon for us women.

➢ Water filters filter out harmful chlorine and other contaminants in your home, either at the shower head or faucets or both. A whole-house water filtration system will take care of your entire home.

➢ If you like fragrance in your laundry, put a few drops of lavender essential oil in the bottle of fragrance-free detergent and on dryer sheets.

Detox To Do:

___ See about taking some time off work for the first week or two.

___ Stock up on all the supplements you will need.

___ If you will be doing the salt baths, stock up on epsom salts and essential oils, as well as a candy thermometer.

___ Swap out your old chemical-laden cleaning, health and beauty products for all-natural, organic ones. Do it gradually if needed, as budget allows.

___ Rotate your antifungal supplements for maximum effect.

___ Look into installing water filters in your home.

Chapter 3 - Self Care

If you are like me, by this time you are familiar with "self care", meaning that you have sought relief for your symptoms. Just as when you were suffering endlessly with the symptoms of candida overgrowth, now you are suffering, although temporarily, with symptoms of candida overgrowth *elimination*. The two are very similar, as mentioned in Chapter 2. In this chapter I will list some natural ways to find relief during your detox for various areas of the body which are affected by candida overgrowth.

So, let's get right to it, as I know you are probably eager to!

Digestive System

If, like me, your weakest area is your gut, you know the misery it can cause when things aren't right. To make matters worse, having issues in this area can be, well, "lonely". By that I mean you usually don't want to, or can't, be social when you have digestive issues. Having to run to the restroom, having issues with burping and gas, not to mention debilitating abdominal pain, is just not something you want to deal with when you are out on the town, or at a party, etc. Heck it's not something you want to deal with at all, ever!

But you are now finally able to do something about it, and here is where you will find advice on how to find a little relief without taking drugs, which only hurt you in the long run.

The following are the natural treatments I found to work for me. I hope they help you too!

Digestive Enzymes. Take a high quality enzyme with each meal. Enzymes will help you to digest the various foods you eat, such as proteins, carbs, and lactose if you are eating Greek yogurt. If you experience digestive upset frequently, no matter what you eat (because candida has damaged your gut), you will find these symptoms lessened by the use of enzymes taken just before you eat. I use Garden Of Life's Omega-Zyme Ultra. This product contains lactase for dairy, which helps me to digest my Greek yogurt. You will find that a lot of enzyme products do not contain lactase for some reason, and you have to buy that separate. So it's up to you and what you eat on the healing diet....if you don't eat yogurt, you shouldn't be eating any other dairy and would be safe using a product with no lactase.

Probiotics. As mentioned previously, probiotics are a *must* for healing. In fact, they should be a part of your daily supplement regimen for the rest of your life if you want to maintain the good health you have once you are done with the healing phase of this plan. Flooding your gut with the beneficial bacteria it needs will go a long way in not only your healing, but your overall health as well. When your gut isn't right, your overall health isn't right. An overgrowth of candida cannot happen in a gut that has the proper amount of good bacteria. I even take an extra capsule if I'm having a flare-up. So they can be used for prevention and treatment. Of course, with my digestive system being my worst area, I spare no expense and use Garden Of Life's Primal Defense Ultra probiotics.

Activated Charcoal. Activated charcoal helps to remove toxins and gas in the gut, and also neutralizes odor if you have issues with gas. You may want to carry this must-have supplement with you at all times during your detox.

Peppermint Oil. Another must-have during detox, and any time a flare-up occurs. Peppermint oil is not only an antifungal, it has very powerful anti-gas properties and will actually dissipate gas (as opposed to forcing it out), relieving bloating and pain within minutes. There are two ways you can use this wonderful oil:

1. **Capsules.** Along with the activated charcoal, a peppermint capsule can go a long way to calm a distressed tummy. A lot of over the counter stomach remedies, like Pepto Bismol, even use peppermint in their formulas. Why not get the real thing without all the other mysterious ingredients? Just be sure to get enteric-coated capsules, as peppermint oil is strong

31

stuff and you will not enjoy burping it up if it breaks open in your stomach. An enteric-coated capsule will get past the stomach acids so it can get to your intestines where it's needed. I use Swanson's Peppermint Oil Combination Enteric Coated, from Swansonvitamins.com.

2. **Essential Oil.** Another way you can use peppermint oil is topically. It may sound strange, but you can actually rub this oil right on your abdomen with a cotton ball, and it will soak through to take care of gas, bloating and pain. In fact, I personally have found this to work quicker and better than capsules, but I often use both together for maximum effectiveness. I use it full strength, but if you find this too strong, you can dilute it in a carrier oil such as grapeseed oil. You can find these oils online or at your local health store.

Curcumin. This comes from the spice turmeric, and is known to be effective for treating pain and inflammation. During detox, I used this as an alternative to ibuprofen.

Magnesium. I mostly used magnesium to treat abdominal pain, as it had a calming effect, both to my gut and to me. I would recommend taking this only at bedtime, as it will help you relax and fall asleep.

Heating pad. Also a staple item when treating abdominal pain. Like magnesium, the heat (at a low setting) will help to relax and calm your abdominal area, and you. I also recommend using this at bedtime, but just remember to turn it off before you fall asleep, or better yet buy one that has an auto shut-off feature.

Lastly, I will list here the very method I used that worked very well for me when I had digestive distress (and still use if I ever have flare-ups):

1. **Take the following supplements** (if I don't list an actual brand, any brand will do):
    - 1 - Primal Defense Ultra probiotic
    - 1 - Swanson's Enteric Coated Peppermint capsule
    - 4 - 260 mg activated charcoal
    - 1 - 400 mg magnesium
    - 1 - 800 mg curcumin

2. **Rub peppermint oil onto abdomen with a cotton ball.**

2. **Place a heating pad on abdomen. Adjust heat to your own comfort level.**

4. **Rest quietly and avoid stress.**

Ears

Do you have a deep down itch inside your ears that you just cannot reach? If you do, you would agree that it's maddening. I did not realize this was candida, but in my research uncovered that candida could indeed cause this. I have had this problem for literally decades, without knowing what caused it. Of course, as my overall health worsened, so did this.

In fact, in the few years before I rid myself of the candida overgrowth, I developed a form of tinnitus. I did not realize it was tinnitus until I looked it up and learned about it. Mine was apparently a rare type where I had a painful clicking and ticking in my right ear. It felt like something was tightening or cramping inside and I would hear the clicking noise. Once I was cleansed of the candida, lo and behold I never had that issue again! One of the wonderful things I discovered while doing this plan was that I resolved a few health issues that I did not even imagine were caused by the candida.

Treating the ears is as simple as doing the diet and detox, and then using the ear drops every night before bed. Personally I found the best time to do this was right after my bath.

You can use the following to treat your ears:
- Wally's Famous Ear Oil, which I found at my local health store. Follow directions on the bottle.

- Coconut oil – apply a pea-sized amount to ear opening and let it melt into the ear canal.
- Hydrogen peroxide – using a dropper, apply 10 drops into each ear.

Here is the method I used:
- Lay down on your left side while treating your right ear (to keep the oil in), while reading a book or watching TV, then flip over to drain, and then do the other ear.
- Do about 20 minutes to a half hour per ear.
- Keep cotton swabs on hand to swab out residual oil.

At first, when your ears still have a lot of yeast in them, you may experience intense itching, tingling or warm sensation in your ears as you treat them. Try to resist the temptation to drain the oil prematurely so you can get a swab in there to scratch that itch. I would press and rub the area right behind my ear lobe to find a little relief, so I could keep the oil in. As the yeast gets less and less over the course of your treatment, you will have little to no discomfort. That's when you know you have healthy ears once again!

Scalp & Skin

Itchy, flakey scalp. I also had this for decades without realizing what caused it, or that dandruff was actually caused by yeast overgrowth on the scalp. In my research, I also learned about scalp psoriasis. But

I am only addressing the dandruff caused by yeast here, as psoriasis is a different issue.

There are many natural products that are effective against dandruff. The same herbs and oils that are effective in supplement form can also be found in a bottle of organic shampoo and conditioner. Some ingredients to look for include:

- Coconut Oil
- Olive Leaf Extract
- Tea Tree Oil
- Eucalyptus Oil
- Peppermint Oil

My shampoo and conditioner of choice are Desert Essence Coconut shampoo and conditioner. When I first used these, my scalp almost burned as the yeast was killed off. If you experience this, don't panic. It's a good thing! Like with your ears, as the excess yeast is killed off, you will not experience any more discomfort.

As for your skin, you may have various rashes on your body caused by yeast. Us ladies commonly have yeast rashes under the breasts. Any place that is warm and gets moist from sweating can develop a yeast rash. Keep a small jar of coconut oil in your medicine cabinet and apply coconut oil to any rashes, both after a shower in the morning or sweat bath in the evening. In fact, any of the oils listed above for your scalp are also effective against skin rashes.

Vaginal / Anal

To treat these sensitive areas, I found gentle ingredients are the best. Two treatments to use:

- For vaginal yeast infection, keep a separate small tub of plain Greek yogurt, dip a tampon to coat the top 1" with yogurt and insert for at least 4 hours. You may even do this before bed. Be sure to keep the yogurt refrigerated to keep the probiotics alive and well.
- For anal itch, rub coconut oil around and just inside the anus. It helps to keep a small jar of coconut oil at your work in case you need to use it. This problem can be as maddening as ear itch so you will want ready relief wherever you are.

Sinuses

In the past, I had missed a few days of work due to sinus issues. If you find that you are prone to sinus infections, especially when the weather is wet and humid, you mostly likely have candida overgrowth in your sinus cavities. While antibiotics may seem to solve the problem now, they will only make things worse in the long run, and even cause your sinuses to be more prone than ever to infections.

While you are detoxing, you will probably experience a strange smell in your sinuses, drainage that seems to go on forever, headaches and just some of the symptoms you had when you had an infection. But now you know that it's because your sinuses are being cleansed, and that there's light at the end of the tunnel!

Here are the natural supplements and methods I used to successfully treat my sinuses during detox. I also use these if I ever have a flare-up (which is now a rare occurrence).

- Garlic Capsules – 200 mg, two capsules after each meal (at least 3x per day). Be sure not to take these on an empty stomach as it will probably cause stomach upset.

- Pau D'Arco tea. You can find this tea at your local health store. The brand I use is Traditional Medicinals. Hold the mug of steaming tea close to your nose and inhale the steam a few times before each sip. Pau D'Arco is an effective natural antifungal.

- Olive Leaf Extract – 500 – 750 mg, one capsule taken with the garlic capsules. Olive Leaf Extract is yet another herb with powerful antifungal properties.

- Steam. Boil some water on the stove and hold a towel over your head as you bend over to inhale the steam. This helps to loosen mucus and for your sinuses to drain.

Self Care Tips

➢ Pack a little "to-go" bag with your must-have supplements to take with you when you go out (if for example you experience digestive distress while out to dinner). I used to keep mine in a small tote bag that I'd grab before heading out the door. Trust me when I say you will not regret doing this! Some good staples to start with are peppermint oil capsules, activated charcoal, small jar of coconut oil, garlic capsules and digestive enzymes. I even used to pack a plastic baggie with a small bottle of peppermint oil and a cotton ball in case I needed the "heavy ammo".

➢ Keeping a humidifier or vaporizer next to your bed at night will help your nasal passages from drying out and becoming irritated and inflamed, especially in the wintertime. Put a little eucalyptus oil in the vapor cup if it has one.

➢ If you are going to spend some time outdoors working in the yard, you may want to consider wearing a dust mask. Especially if you are going to be down near the ground or raking leaves, because mold spores being released as you work will aggravate your sinuses.

➢ You may want to invest in a saline nasal irrigation kit. This helps to keep your sinuses clear of any contaminants like mold or pollen and also to help keep them clean as the yeast dies off. Especially helpful during allergy season.

> Keeping mold in your home to a minimum will not only help your sinuses but your overall health and that of your family.

Self Care To Do:

___ Make your "to-go" bag.

___ Set up your "ear care" station by your bedside – ear oil, cotton swabs and a good book.

___ Visit your local drug store to purchase a heating pad, humidifier and nasal irrigation kit.

___ If you aren't sure which shampoo to start with for treating your scalp, put a few drops of tea tree and eucalyptus oil in your existing shampoo to help make it more therapeutic.

Chapter 4 - Stress Management

Keeping stress to a minimum during your healing is of utmost importance, as stress can literally change your body's chemistry in a negative way and limit its ability to heal. In fact, chronic, continuous stress may be one of the causes of your candida overgrowth.

Now I know how hard it can be to not feel stress when you are in a stressful situation. The only thing I have found to help me in those cases is prayer and deep breathing, so I stay more calm. I have a tendency to speak my feelings as I'm feeling them, and it only makes things worse if the feelings are stressful. So those two things help calm me down enough so I can speak calmly and not say negative things even though I have a raging storm inside of me. Soon the storm passes and I am so glad I handled the situation well in the end.

What also really helps is to limit the chances of stressful situations to begin with. This means more "down time" or "me time" especially if you are a busy mom or just someone who is always in demand by others. Get your spouse's assistance here, or even your children if they are old enough to do some things themselves. If you are a single parent, look into bartering with your friends and family (they take your kids one day, you take theirs another or do another type of favor for them). Get creative, it's worth it! This also means saying "no" more often to social commitments or special requests by others, or to getting involved at your church or work if it is not totally necessary.

Choose your battles. If you feel some things are more stressful than others, then avoid those things and instead do the things that will not have a negative affect on your healing. It may even mean cutting back on existing commitments. For people who love to be plugged in and involved, or be helpful and available to others, this may not be an easy task. But if you tell yourself it's just temporary so you can maximize your healing, it may not seem so bad.

You might even want to let others know, depending on your relationships, that you are treating a health issue and need to limit yourself for now. I did this and nobody ever thought it was strange. Everyone who is reasonable will understand, and maybe even admire you for what you are doing. In the end, when you are much healthier, you will be able to jump back in and handle everything with much less stress than you used to because now you feel so much better and stronger, both physically, mentally and emotionally!

Of course, there are natural supplements that help you in this area also. Here are some I recommend and have used:

- Homeopathic "calms" (type "calm" in the search field in Swansonvitamins.com to see all the different varieties. I used Swanson Homeopathy calms).
- Magnesium
- GABA (helps your brain)
- Valerian Root (relaxes your body and mind, wonderful stuff if you don't mind the odor!)

Stress Management Tips

> Your sweat baths can be a very peaceful "me time" you look forward to. Read a good, positive, calming and uplifting book or magazine while soaking.

> Try doing Qi-Gong or gentle yoga. For Qi-Gong, I recommend www.exercisetoheal.com.

> Spend time in meditation and/or prayer.

> Go for walks at a relaxed pace, listen to audio books or relaxing music.

> Indulge in a professional massage.

> Keep a journal. Sometimes writing it all out helps clear the mind and eliminate stress.

> Limit your commitments.

> Pay attention to the things, places or people that make you feel peaceful, and get more of these into your life. At the same time, weed out the negative.

Stress Management To Do:

___ Stock up on calming supplements and keep some at work or where ever you feel most stressed.

___ Incorporate stress-relief type activities into your lifestyle, such as walks, Qi-gong, yoga, prayer, and saying "no" to too many commitments.

___ Set a basket of good books or magazines by your bath tub.

___ Buy a blank book or journal at your local book store.

Chapter 5 - Sleep

Just as important as diet and stress-management, getting good quality sleep is essential to your healing. In this chapter will be ways to maximize sleep as much as possible during the healing phase.

First a couple of basic goals to shoot for: get to bed by 11 pm latest, and aim for 7-8 hours of sleep per night. Getting to bed by 11 is one thing, but getting 7 to 8 hours of sleep may be a struggle.

Here are some supplements that are helpful for sleep. You will recognize a few of them from previous chapters:

- Valerian Root – as needed
- Magnesium – 250 - 400 mg
- Evening Primrose Oil – 1300 mg daily
- Melatonin – 3 - 9 mg

I take the Evening Primrose Oil with my dinner each day. Its effect on sleep is more indirect, so there is no advantage in taking it right at bedtime. Basically, EPO helps balance hormones (mostly for us ladies), which in turn helps us sleep. The others more quickly relax you and help you to fall asleep.

If you wake in the middle of the night, you can take another melatonin or a couple valerian roots to help you fall back asleep. Unlike with most OTC sleep aids, you will not feel drowsy in the morning from any of these supplements.

Sleep Tips:

- ➢ The body cooling down activates melatonin, so take your bath right before bed.

- ➢ Keep your bedroom between 60° and 68° for optimal sleep.

- ➢ No TV/Computer before bed (ideally, read quietly).

- ➢ Shut off all light sources, If possible, shut off all electronics/wifi, etc., and invest in light blocking curtains to make the bedroom as dark as possible. At the least, wear a sleep mask to block light.

- ➢ Use a white-noise machine if you are a light sleeper.

- ➢ Do not drink any liquids 2 hours before bed (except for when you need to take sleep aids).

- ➢ If insomnia is a real problem, ask your boss if you can flex your work hours temporarily, such as coming in an hour or two later. An understanding boss may agree to a temporary change for health-related reasons, not to mention having a more productive employee not prone to making mistakes due to lack of sleep!

Sleep To Do:

___ Stock up on Valerian Root and Melatonin supplements to keep at your bedside.

___ Add Evening Primrose Oil to your daily supplement program if you are female.

___ Get a thermometer for your bedroom.

___ If noise wakes you up often, invest in a white noise machine.

___ Hang light-blocking curtains or blinds in your bedroom or wear a sleep mask.

Chapter 6 - Healing Phase:
A Day In The Life

In this chapter I will put together all of the information discussed so far for the healing phase into an actual real-life model for you to use as a daily guide.

As mentioned earlier, the more strictly you follow the healing phase plan, the quicker and more complete will be your recovery from candida overgrowth. The healing phase will last 3 to 6 months, depending on how strictly you follow it. It may even last longer than 6 months.

So let's look at a "day in the life" of someone who is strictly following their plan. This is just an example to model your healing phase after. It may seem overwhelming, but if you take it one day at a time it will become second nature. NOTE: this model involves working at a full time job as part of your "day". If your schedule differs, or if you take a week or two off work when you start the plan (recommended), simply adjust this to fit your situation.

Morning

- Upon waking, take the following supplements:
  - Probiotic
  - Antifungal such as Fungal Defense (cycle every 2 weeks)
  - Fiber

- Say prayers/meditate.

- Do a short Qi-Gong routine to start the day relaxed, peaceful and centered.

- Take a shower with your new filter installed that eliminates chlorine and other harmful chemicals. Use your organic body wash, shampoo and conditioners.

- Brush your teeth with your organic, flouride-free toothpaste.

- Apply your organic body lotion and aluminum-free deodorant.

- Put on your all natural mineral make-up.

- Get dressed in clothes washed in organic free & clear laundry detergent.

- Pack your candida diet meals and supplements to take to work for the day. Use a small cooler if you don't have a refrigerator at work to keep it in.

- Take your "self-care to-go kit" to work with you, just in case!

- Prepare your sugar-free whey protein shake in your blender bottle, add stevia to taste. Take it with you in the car to sip on the way to work. Be sure to take an enzyme right beforehand. Breakfast...done!

- After breakfast, take the following supplements:
    - 2000 mg Vitamin D3 (for immune system)
    - 1 Oregano Oil capsule (enteric coated)
    - 1 Milk Thistle
    - 1 Adrenal Stress End
    - 1 Olive Leaf Extract

- The work day is getting a little crazy, so take a calms or a valerian root to take the edge off the stress if you feel it creeping up. Take deep breaths, take a walk!

- Time for your mid-morning snack of 1 cup Greek yogurt sweetened with stevia.

- Your sinuses are killing you, so you take two 1000 mg garlic capsules after each snack and meal today (eight total), and you enjoy a mug of Pau D'Arco tea.

- Take the following supplements with your lunch:
  - 1 Omega-zyme (enzyme)
  - 2000 mg Vitamin D3
  - Probiotic
  - Whole Food Multivitamin
  - 1000 mg Fish Oil
  - 1 Adrenal Stress End

Afternoon

- Thank goodness you purposely left all your change and dollar bills at home, as you were mighty tempted when you walked by the vending machines today!

- You have a maddening itch "down there", so you grab your little vial of coconut oil from your to-go kit and head to the restroom. Once applied, you have relief and can get back to work.

- It's 3 pm and you crave a cold soda, so you grab your flavored sparkling water, add stevia (and liquid caffeine, though this should be limited during the healing phase) to make a refreshing, healthy, cold and fizzy beverage. Or, you brew some flavored green tea, add stevia and pour over ice. You feel great that you avoided the junk! Battle won!

- People watch you mixing your healthy concoctions with curiosity. Brag about what you are doing! You are watching your health and what you put into your body, and that is admirable! Over time, you may notice people around you becoming more health-conscious as they see you getting healthier and thinner.....it's contagious!

- It's 4 pm so you enjoy your mid-afternoon snack of 2-3 hard boiled eggs with sea salt.

- You've talked to your boss today about changing your hours as you have really been struggling with insomnia. Your boss agrees to a trial period and if it did not affect your work or the company negatively, you could stay on it as long as needed. You feel a big sense of relief, that finally you may start getting that sleep you need so much.

- It's 5 pm and time to go home. You quickly review your day in your mind, and you are very proud of yourself so far at sticking with your plan and even getting your work hours changed so you can hopefully get that sleep you need. Those calms really helped keep you from getting stressed out today, too, and because you handled the day so well, you look better to those around you and your boss. The bonus: your health is better for it too!

- It's time for dinner. You've made a wonderful meal that is on-plan and that you love, so it's not a sacrifice. You may even share it with your family so you won't have to cook two dinners, and you feel good knowing that they are eating healthy.

- Take the following supplements with dinner:
  - 1 Omega-zyme (enzyme)
  - Whole Food Multivitamin
  - 1000 mg Fish Oil
  - 1300 mg Evening Primrose Oil
  - Antifungal such as Fungal Defense (cycle every 2 weeks)

Evening

- After dinner, you go for a short, leisurely walk.

- Once back from your walk, you notice you need to do some weeding. You make sure to put on a dust mask to avoid breathing in any mold spores.

- After yardwork, you do some more Qi-Gong to help your digestive system and stress.

- It's about 2 hours before bedtime, so now it's time for your nightly self-care routine. As your bath fills (with the candy thermometer floating in the water to get the right temp), you check to be sure you have a book, ear oil and cotton swabs on your nightstand, along with a vaporizer with eucalyptus oil in the cup next to your bed. You have staged your nasal irrigation kit by the sink. You also have a magazine, epsom salts and essential oils by the tub, along with a couple towels. You add 5 drops each of lavender, tea tree and eucalyptus oils to the bath water, along with 2 cups of epsom salts.

- After a good sweat in your bath for about 30 minutes, you are really feeling the detox, as you are feeling very tired. The ring around the tub at the waterline tells you that you have gotten rid of some toxins! You are looking forward to the times when you feel refreshed after your baths, but that will be when you are mostly detoxed.

- After drying off, it's time for the nasal irrigation. You especially felt the need for this as your sinuses have been bothering you as the yeast dies off, so the irrigation will help remove the dead yeast as well.

- You brush your teeth with your flouride-free toothpaste once again.

- You notice some pain in your gut since your bath, so you take activated charcoal, magnesium and curcumin capsules, rub some peppermint oil on your belly and grab the heating pad.

- You go over to your bedside and turn on the vaporizer.

- You lay down on your side and place the heating pad over your belly.

- Time for the ears. You put ear oil drops in one ear, grab your book and relax for about 30 minutes. It's so itchy at first, but you soldier through it and it calms down after a few minutes. You flip over to empty that ear and treat the other ear. All in all, this routine can take up to 1 hour, but it's so worth it.

- Time for sleep. Your belly is feeling better, so that will help. Even though you feel sleepier as your body cooled from the sweat bath, you take a valerian root and/or a melatonin for insurance (they can be taken together). You have made sure the room will be as dark as possible by turning off all sources of light and using room-darkening curtains and shades. You check your new room thermometer to make sure the temperature of the room is between 60° and 68°. You have turned off your heating pad. Lastly, you feel more relaxed just knowing you have a couple of extra hours to catch up on any lost sleep if you wake up in the middle of the night, since your new work hours start tomorrow.

- You wake at 2 am, like so many other nights. Knowing that you won't be able to sleep until about 4 am doesn't bother you as much now though, due to the fact that you can sleep in to catch up. This alone helps you to relax and get back to sleep quicker. Plus you know that as time goes on, your insomnia should be reduced greatly or go away completely once you are healed.

Morning Again

- It's 9 am and time to get up. You fell back asleep around 3:30 am with the help of some more valerian root and melatonin, and now that you reclaimed the lost sleep time, you feel refreshed and ready to do it all over again today. Then you smile because you are one day closer to being cured and fully healed!

Chapter 7 - Maintenance

It's been at least a few months, and you feel you are pretty much healed. Your energy is high, steady and lasting through the day, with no slumps. You are back to your normal work hours and having only the rare night of insomnia. You don't feel depressed anymore. If you are a 40-something woman, your hormones are balanced, with no more hot flashes or PMS symptoms. All your digestive and sinus symptoms have completely disappeared, and you are amazed at how great you feel, and just how bad off you were before.

If you have been good about sticking to your healing phase plan and have little to no symptoms remaining, and it's been at least 3 months, you can feel safe about *gently* reintroducing the forbidden foods to your diet and reducing the antifungal supplements to a maintenance level, all the while closely monitoring your body's reactions with each reintroduction.

The earliest indications of yeast overgrowth reoccuring would mostly likely be in the digestive system (bloating, gas, IBS), vaginal yeast infections and sinus issues (congestion, headaches, infection). If you tried a sugary dessert one day and experienced digestive upset and a sinus headache afterwards, you know it was probably too much too soon. Or maybe that one dessert did not cause any problems. So the next day, you had something else with a lot of sugar in it, and then something else the day after that.

Then suddenly you had symptoms.

That is what happened with me, it was more of a cumulative effect over a few days. I learned that I had to keep my sugar intake of over 5 grams down to only a couple of days per week, and I could not ingest something that had over 15 grams all at once or I had immediate flare-ups. My first indicators were digestive problems, itchy ears and sinus headaches. This lasted for a good eight months to a year. It's been almost 2 years since I went on my healing phase plan and I'm finally able to eat "normally" without fear of flare-ups. By "normally" I mean 24 grams per day without any issues.

However, I still try to keep the sugar low as much as possible, for obvious health reasons. I have for the most part changed my diet for the better, and now I can enjoy the occasional treat without getting sick for days afterwards!

So don't be discouraged if your post-healing maintenance phase lasts as long as one year. Stick with your daily probiotics and treat flare-ups with the strict diet and supplements that you used during the healing phase until they have cleared, then go back to the maintenance plan with the knowledge you now have about what your body's present limits are. The reintroduction period can last for months, so you will have to be patient. You certainly don't want to lose all the progress you've made, so take your time, listen to your body, and act accordingly.

Maintenance Tips:

➤ Start with adding 5 grams of sugar more than what you were taking in on the healing phase (which should be about 10 grams) and monitor your body's reactions, if any. Cut back to the healing phase plan if you experience flare-ups.

➤ As with sugar, add forbidden foods back to your diet one group at a time, and monitor your body's reactions. Digestive issues would most likely be the first flare-up you have with foods, even while you are eating them. If no flare-ups, continue to eat the food in moderation. If and when you have a flare-up, cut back accordingly until symptoms clear.

➤ Sweat baths should now only be done when treating flare-ups, to help the body more quickly detox and heal.

➤ Strong antifungal supplements that are formulated specifically to clear candida overgrowth, like Fungal Defense, should now only be taken for flare-ups.

➤ Supplements like oregano oil and olive leaf extract may still be taken daily for up to 6 months to a year after the healing phase to help minimize the occurence and intensity of any flare-ups.

Maintenance To Do:

___ Avoid antibiotics if at all possible!

___ Add forbidden foods back to your diet one group at a time, and monitor your body's reactions.

___ Continue with your new healthier lifestyle of water filters, natural cleaners, organic lotions and bath/shower products, etc.

___ Continue to keep your sugar intake as low as possible as a rule, and keep eating as organically as possible.

Chapter 8 - Encouragement

I just wanted to wrap up this book with a few words of encouragement. Whether you've read through this book before beginning your journey, or you have been living out the steps as you read, I want to encourage you to keep going and hang in there, you are worth it!

You find that it feels good to be taking care of yourself and doing what is good for your body, and the icing on the cake is your body rewarding you with more energy, less (or no) aches and pains, and just overall better health. When you first start feeling that "better" feeling, you will pause and think "Wow, I feel GREAT right now!" If you haven't been well in a long time, you may have forgotten how it feels to be healthy, and when you start feeling that way, it will really help keep you motivated.

Our bodies were created to heal as long as we give them what they need to do this miraculous thing called healing. You may even notice bonuses like illnesses and chronic conditions that are suddenly gone, that you did not realize were caused by the candida overgrowth. Ladies, those hot flashes will most likely become history, and stay that way as long as you keep your sugar intake low. Your body will just be in balance, and you will feel the way you are supposed to feel: *healthy!*

Lastly, I also want to encourage you to visit my blog at cureyourcandida.blogspot.com. There you will find a variety of information for and about the treatment and cure of candida overgrowth. Because I am ever finding new information about so many things that affect candida, I feel it's important to share my findings in my blog. Be sure to stop in and say hello!

About The Author

Linda Shaw lives in southeast Michigan with her family. She enjoys writing, vacationing in beautiful northern Michigan, decorating, cooking, nature, loves animals and caring for the family pets, boating, classic car shows and cruises. She is also passionate about natural health and continually finding ways to live naturally by researching nutrition, learning about natural remedies and making natural homemade products.

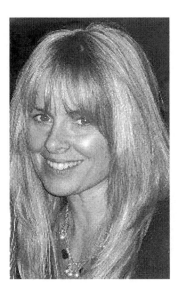

After years of declining health, Linda went about thoroughly researching candida overgrowth and put together a completely natural self-treatment plan. Six months and 20 lost pounds later, she realized that her plan worked better than she had ever dreamed.

Inspired, she wrote "The Candida Remedy" so she could share her success, and has also published the journal she kept while healing from the candida overgrowth, titled "Diary Of A Candida Sufferer: A Personal Journey Back To Health".

Linda hopes to publish more books in the future.